The Link Between Amanita muscaria and Marijuana

*This book does not recommend consuming ANY drugs! This book is for documentation and research purposes only.

Introduction

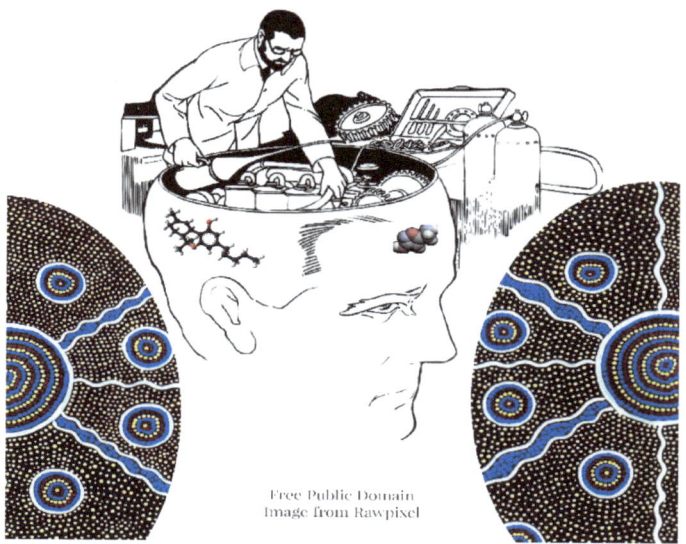

Free Public Domain
Image from Rawpixel

Well….. where do I even begin? If you don't
know, don't worry. That's simply a rhetorical
question to help jump-start the book. I always
struggle to find the proper words to begin, but
nevertheless here we are. So this is my third
small book on Amanita muscaria, with my other
two being "The Legal Magic Mushrooms of
North America: A Study of the Amanita
muscaria Varieties" and "Amanita muscaria:
The Ritualistic Magic Mushrooms". Now both
titles are rather long, yet also rather self
explanatory — so I won't go into them in great
detail here.

However, I will mention that each book serves its own purpose in the wild world of magic mushrooms. The first is about the types of Amanita muscaria varieties that grow wild in North America, namely Amanita muscaria var. guessowii. I detail the growing habitat, possibilities of cultivation, legality, effects and so on. The second book focuses more on the history (mostly in North America) of the mushrooms and their ritualistic uses. With both citing studies and previous writings regarding the fungi.

But, with this book I aim to tackle something that I've already briefly touched on in my first and second book about the mushrooms, and that is the mixture of marijuana with Amanita muscaria (more specifically the psychoactive ingredients Delta-9 and muscimol) which seems to produce effects that can't be found when both substances are used individually. So there is some sort of a link between the two, a synergistic link. I think the best way to describe it, is likening the process to how the indigenous brew ayahuasca, a famous hallucinogenic drink.

This is done with a combination of different plants and trees, creating a unique psychedelic experience. I've always enjoyed mixing drugs, so the process of mixing marijuana and Amanita muscaria mushrooms came rather naturally to me. Much like "hippie-flipping" with LSD and mushrooms (or maybe candyflipping LSD+MDMA), either way, you get the idea. At first, I smoked marijuana with the mushrooms and documented the effects. Then I ate some on a separate day, but I didn't think the "buzz" was so great eating them (with no marijuana included this time).

Then, I saw these gummies online for sale by a few different companies and they were mixed with cannabinoids. Now this produced the strong psychedelic effect that I was looking for, similar to when I smoked it combined but even more powerful. Many of these online retailers will sell them in a package of 10, with each gummy containing something like 350-500mg of Amanita muscaria, and 15-50mg or so of either Delta-8, 9, 10, 11, HHC, THC-A etc. However, combined with Delta-9 seems to be by far the most popular.

So, my experience at first was sort of hit-or-miss is what I'm trying to say when I experienced the mushrooms by themselves. But the gummies mixed with cannabinoids were a success every single time. But why could that be? I wondered about this, and then I began researching. I've read countless claims from various people who ingested Amanita muscaria gummies, and for lack of a better term, they were bummed out. Many people felt ripped off and felt like those who recommended the mushrooms, have misled them. Some people have even gone as far as to call these magic mushrooms useless.

But, I noticed one major detail in the vast majority of these stories — and that is the fact that most of them had the exact same thing in common — which was there was no delta-8, 9, 10, 11, HHC, THC-A... nothing. So what exactly is happening? Well, I fully intend on documenting and discussing the entirety of this very complex link between Amanita muscaria mushrooms and marijuana throughout this book, so I truly hope you enjoy reading it as much as I've enjoyed writing it! With that being said, let's begin.

Part One

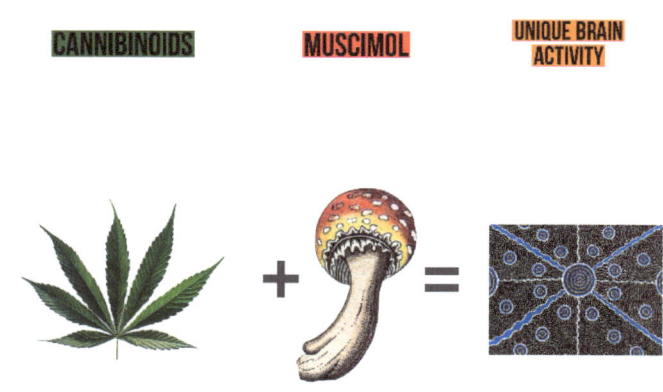

Free Public Domain
Images from Rawpixel

With no marijuana compounds to be found, could that be the key? As I sit here today, I can say with absolute certainty that it is. So psychedelic enthusiasts, rejoice! Because I'm about to break it all down for you, and I'm excited as I write this so hopefully you will be just as thrilled to read it. But, rest assured you won't have to just take my word for it either. As I will be providing plenty of hard evidence to back my claims.

So my first example that I will present, is (as far as I'm aware) the first documented study that shows the synergistic relationship between marijuana cannabinoids and muscimol. The study I'm referring to, is titled *"Drugs which stimulate or facilitate central GABAergic transmission interact synergistically with delta-9-tetrahydrocannabinol to produce marked catalepsy in mice"*. This article was published by the National Library of Medicine [NLM] in 1988. Within the article was this important piece of information; "only (+)-bicuculline reduced the interactions of THC with muscimol and cis(Z)-flupentixol".

This article appeared just 3 years prior to the next one that I will highlight, which was also published by the NLM in 1991, titled; "Drugs which stimulate or facilitate central cholinergic transmission interact synergistically with delta-9-tetrahydrocannabinol to produce marked catalepsy in mice". So this incredible discovery was made more than 30 years ago, yet somehow today it's rarely mentioned — which is odd with so much renewed interest with psychedelics. But that's not to say that drug enthusiasts haven't taken notice, as I've previously mentioned I'm hardly the first to discuss this relationship.

Another example was published in 1995, in the European Journal of Pharmacology article titled; "Effect of DELTA(9)-Tetrahydrocannabinol on circling in rats induced by itranagiral muscimol administration". Within the article was this conclusion; "synergism between Delta(9)-tetrahydrocannabinol and muscimol can occur". The author(s) would later mention an increased "excitatory" effect. Furthermore, I previously mentioned how muscimol was first isolated from Amanita muscaria (actually possibly Amanita pantherina, brown caps) in 1964, well, one year later in 1965 was when muscimol was first synthesized.

So with the knowledge of these government (tax-payer) funded studies, it's really not that much of a coincidence that these products are often sold as one (mixed together) whether it's gummies or vapes, and sometimes even a beverage. The knowledge was apparently out there for those who knew where to look. I published my second short book about Amanita muscaria mushrooms [Amanita muscaria: The Ritualistic Magic Mushrooms] in late May, 2023 (with my first book on the topic published in 2022).

Within the latter, I discuss my own personal smoke blend I enjoy, being Amanita muscaria mushrooms mixed with "tobacco" and "marijuana". I discuss how the mixture of marijuana and Amanita muscaria served as one of the "coolest hallucinogenic cigarettes I've ever tried" and I would further mention that "the gummies that are infused with Delta-9 and muscimol" are "the ideal combination".

I also mentioned that "The drug [muscimol] will have different effects when mixed with other drugs". The "other drugs" I briefly discussed on the page just before [page 27 to be exact] was Delta-9 specifically. Then, more than a month after I published the book [May, 2023], an article was published by "The Calm Leaf", and they too highlighted the possibility of the same connection. Again, this isn't a discovery either of us made, this was already established in documented studies from the 1980s and 1990s.

Nevertheless, The Calm Leaf published an article on July 1, 2023 titled; "Do Amanita Mushrooms React Differently with Cannabinoids I've Taken?". But within the article the author writes; "there has been no research on the relationship between amanita muscaria (or, more specifically, muscimol), and cannabinoids". Well, that's just the author's opinion, and I will simply say that I respectfully disagree. As I've previously highlighted, and will continue to highlight throughout my books, there has been plenty of research on the relationship between muscimol and cannabinoids. So with that being said, let's continue.

Muscimol molecule

Delta-9 Molecule

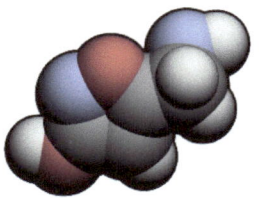 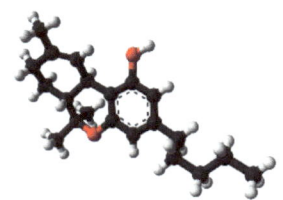

Free Public Domain
Image
Muscimol3d.png
Original file

When I say there has been "plenty of research", I should clarify that I mean that in the loosest of terms, and only in regards to having enough proof to form a conclusion. I'm not saying there has been enough research done on muscimol, or cannabinoids for that matter, let alone the two combined. I'm simply saying enough research has been done to show the two form a synergistic relationship. This is actually very similar to how Amanita muscaria mushrooms grow symbiotically, as they are an ectomycorrhizal fungi (forming a give-and-take relationship with specific plants).

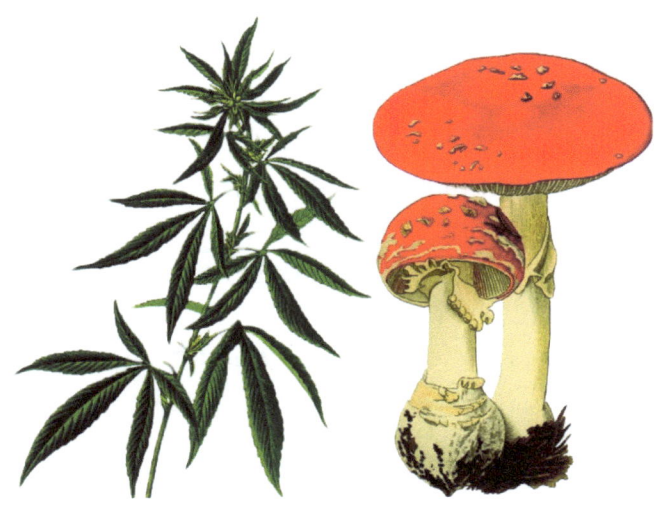

Now, many people have debated how to grow Amanita muscaria mushrooms indoors, as once again they need to connect to the roots of other plants/trees in order to form a symbiotic relationship which benefits both parties. On a website called "Shroomery" I saw a user ask about the possibility of Amanita muscaria forming that relationship with the roots of a marijuana plant (which is an interesting thought if nothing else). I like the idea of that, along with what I've previously written about some sort of protoplast fusion where you basically merge the mushroom with another species (hopefully in order to promote easier cultivating techniques).

I believe Amanita muscaria mushrooms are some of the most under-studied fungi in the world, and without a doubt muscimol is one of the most under-studied drugs. Muscimol was first isolated in 1964, so sixty years ago. Yet, somehow very little is known about it (when compared to other psychedelics). But the relationship that these mushrooms form with plants (both while growing and while consuming them) needs to be examined further.

For example, tobacco also seems to have a synergistic relationship with muscimol, and who knows how another psychedelic may interact, such as psilocybin. Tobacco, in my opinion, has a synergistic relationship with many different drugs. Growing up in Cleveland, it was rather common to roll tobacco with marijuana in a "Philly cigar shell". I've even heard famous people like Joe Rogan discuss the potency when consumed this way.

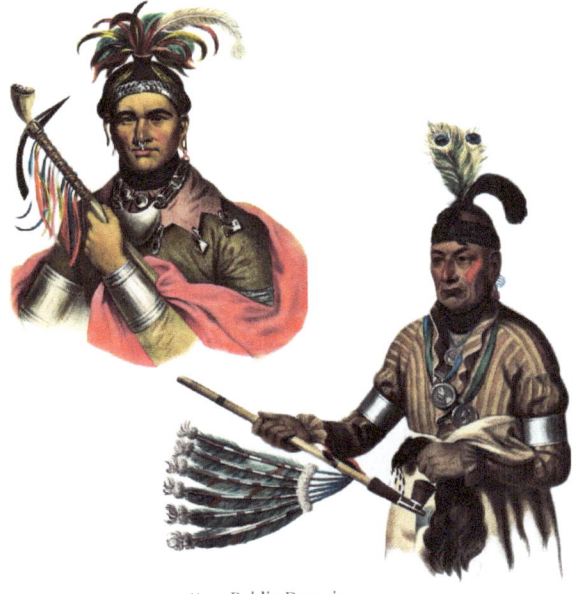

Free Public Domain
Images from Rawpixel

The indigenous people were very big into mixing plants to either smoke and/or eat (as

I've previously mentioned with ayahuasca) and also terms like "kinnikinnick" being an example of said mixing. But today, mixing drugs is typically frowned upon. For an example of this, I can refer to alcohol and pain pills, usually you'll hear people say "don't mix them", and likely rightfully so. But there is a definite advantage to mixing some plants/fungi, but of course caution should always be used (and common sense).

So, I'd like to add something that I've mentioned earlier before continuing, and that is in regards to muscimol and synergistic research. I should clarify that the earliest studies that I cited, was about muscimol forming a synergistic relationship specifically with cannabinoids, not in general. So let me clarify just a bit before proceeding; research has been done earlier about other compounds forming these interactions with muscimol. Notably, studies from 1983 and 1984, both published in the National Library of Medicine (with extremely long titles that I won't include here).

Nevertheless, similar articles were published once again by the NLM, which more-or-less are about synergism and connections to things like memory with obviously another compound(s) being added. So although the research for these three articles are not necessarily related to what I'm discussing, I will spare further detail, but I still found it rather noteworthy to highlight. While I'm on this topic, I have a few more examples before I get back I to the good stuff.

A website named "vidacap" published an article on October 30, 2023 (would've been cooler to wait until Halloween was my first observation, but then again i like weird things) and the article was titled; "Muscimol: Our Guide to Its Effects, Uses, and Potential Benefits". One thing that stood out, at least to me, was the author mentioned something about avoiding "muscimol" and other "GABA-A agonists" which the author highlights included "alcohol".

Similarly, in an article published by "painphysicianjournal" titled; "Combination Opioid Angalesics" the author states "Morphine, muscimol, or baclofen increased both TF latency and CD threshold in a dose-dependent fashion". So, I think it's safe to assume, this compound is magical in many ways. I've even seen an article about combination chemotherapy using muscimol, which was titled "Combination Chemotherapy Extends the Therapeutic Window to 60 Minutes After Stroke" and was published in 2009 by "lieberpub".

In recent studies, muscimol has shown possibilities of relieving pain, itch, nerve damage and a lot more. This compound isolated from these mushrooms that have been around forever, will likely forever change medicine. Wikipedia states that muscimol was "able to significantly alleviate pain in its peak effect, recent studies from 2023 show". While a trial to use muscimol to treat epilepsy was discontinued, according to "European Bioinformatics Institute" in 2020.

In July, 2023, more good news was published by a website named "BlueToadBotanicals" which the author states "Studies suggest that muscimol may stimulate certain receptors in the brain, leading to improved cognitive abilities". Also in 2023, The Korean Journal of Pain published an article "Muscimol as a treatment for nerve injury-related neuropathic pain". In the article, the author discusses muscimol helping the "plasticity" in the "spinal cord". So what we may be looking at here, in my opinion, is a truly magical medicine and ethenogen.

Well…. Look how far we've come since some of the famous mycologists (I won't name names) called Amanita muscaria "one of the most dangerous mushrooms in the world". Well, they are technically poisonous and dangerous, but I also haven't heard much from them as Amanita muscaria products are now beginning to appear in grocery stores in NYC, according to a recently published article titled "Psyched Wellness's Calm, First Legal Amanita Muscaria Extract, Arrives at Pop-up Grocer in NYC" which is dated December 12, 2023.

In my first book about Amanita muscaria from 2022, I told my readers to keep an eye out for the "Canadian start-up company" Psyched Wellness. I saw the moves early on that they were making, and in all honesty I was a bit jealous of not only their imagination, but their funding. I sought out investors too(with no success) but in a different approach, an attempt to cultivate these mushrooms for the first time indoors.

Unfortunately, I couldn't find any takers. Everyone seems to think it's "impossible" to cultivate Amanita muscaria mushrooms indoors, forgetting that the same exact thing was said about cultivating morels (which is now a HUGE booming industry). I'll make a prediction that these mushrooms will be cultivated indoors before 2030. I would be EXTREMELY happy if the first person to do it was me (wishful and perhaps delusional thinking).

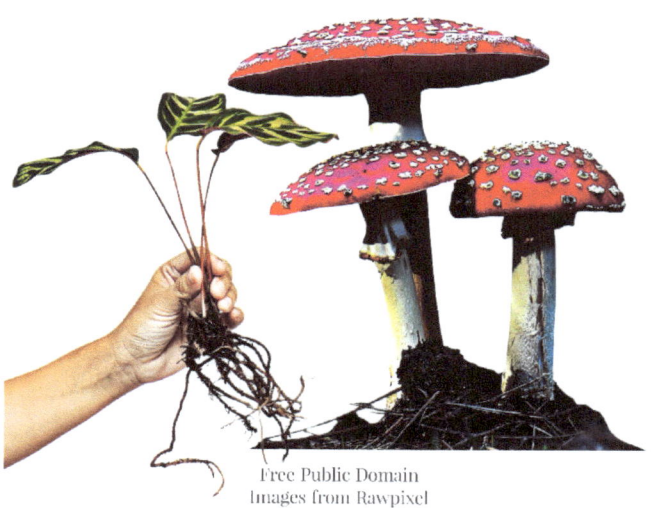

Free Public Domain
Images from Rawpixel

In my second book about Amanita muscaria that I published in 2023, I mentioned that "naturedotcom" published an article in which the author stated; "GABA signaling modulates plant growth". Quite interesting I must say, which is why I've also included it in this book as well. This goes back to the notion that these mushrooms and specific plants not only benefit each other while growing in the ground, but also possibly medicinally and recreationally. Forest ground cover-type plants form a great symbiotic relationship with certain mushrooms, especially a plant like Vinca minor [periwinkle] so it would be interesting to see someone attempt an indoor grow with them. But... this, however, is not what this book is about. You can kindly refer to my previous publications for further in-depth coverage on that topic.

Wikipedia states that the effects of muscimol are "closely comparable to the hallucinogenic side effects" that are produced by "some other drugs", namely "zolpidem". I find this interesting, because I've seen this in generic sleep medication sold online — usually with a stark warning not to mix with alcohol. According to the NLM in an article published in 2002 titled "Binding and neuropharmacological profile of zaleplon, a novel nonbenzodiazepine sedative/hypnotic", the author states zolpidem "produces significant increases in muscimol".

From what I've gathered, zolpidem is part of what's known as the "Z-drugs", similar to the active ingredient in ambien [zolpidem]. So basically this cheap sleeping medication may have some more purpose, but perhaps a bit dangerous to try so best to leave it to the scientific studies. But I could only imagine the absolutely vivid dreams. Well, that seems to be another synergistic relationship, so I'll also include what appears to be another inhibitor, which is (once again according to NLM) taurine. So basically don't ingest taurine (energy drinks or whatever) while using muscimol unless you want the effects somewhat mitigated. This knowledge seems to come from research that dates back to the late 1970s.

Interestingly enough, it should be noted that although taurine negates and/or diminishes the effects of muscimol, taurine also has many benefits by itself. Most notably, many new studies have shown that taurine can in fact "delay aging" and/or better yet, "reverse aging". So please don't dismiss taurine entirely, just because it negates muscimol. Also, who knows taurine may increase the effects of other drugs, much like when I was younger we all would drink orange juice while we took LSD (it sure seemed to work). I've heard of other beverages as well, like grape juice.

Speaking of "grape juice" I've read some conflicting reports of people using grape juice in order to basically isolate muscimol from Amanita muscaria mushrooms. When I Google "grape juice + muscimol" The third result that showed was for a patent; "Method for producing muscimol and/or reducing ibotenic acid from amanita tissue". The article stated that the patent was anticipated to expire in 2033, with it beginning in 2013. Many people liken the grape juice technique of extraction to sacred wine from the Bible, so it's weird to see a patent on it.

Now, back to the LSD talk; according to a website called "pharmacia", "Muscimol and LSD caused a decrease in catecholamines". Catecholamines are basically hormones that are created by adrenal glands. Both drugs all raise serotonin levels. I've personally mixed LSD and muscimol, and had incredible effects that were far superior to either drug taken individually. So, similar to after my experience when combining cannabinoids, I began to research it further.

I also came across others with similar experiences; notably a Reddit user who described the effects as "almost DMT-like". My curiosity got the better of me, so I researched "muscimol combined with MDMA" and found a discouraging article published by NLM in 2008; "Microinjection of muscimol into the dorsomedial hypothalamus suppresses MDMA-evoked sympathetic and behavioral responses". I'm not really sure why that is, maybe due to MDMA being synthetic, but truly who knows.

Muscimol also has a very potent derivative, which is known as "thiomuscimol". Both, pure (or as close to pure as possible) muscimol and "thiomuscimol" have a pretty hefty price tag (at least from what I've gathered by browsing around online). A website that is selling thiomuscimol (as of this writing) in what they advertised as being at least "95% pure", for a price of $270.00 for 5mg. That website is "netascientific", while a separate website named "biosynth" was selling 5mg of thiomuscimol for $330.00.

Part Two

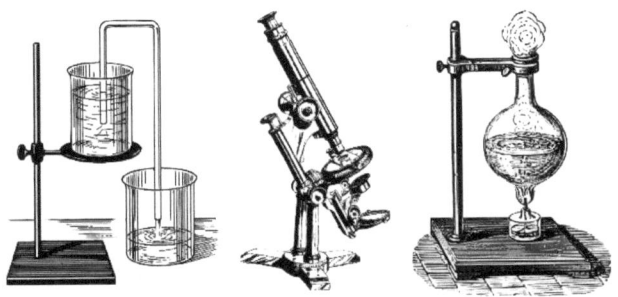

Synthetic muscimol (and pure muscimol for
that matter) can be legally purchased online. In
fact, the knowledge has been widely available
for many years. For example, in 1986 an article
(that can now be found on "sciencedirect") was
published with a title "A convenient synthesis of
muscimol by a 1,3-dipolar cycloaddition
reaction". Within the article, the author
discusses "A simple and large scale synthesis

of muscimol starting from dibromoformaldoxime".

Now most people do not view synthetic drugs as being pure, or as good as the original (and rightfully so), but of course that's addressing synthetic drugs in a very loose manner. I'm not personally against the idea of ingesting synthetic drugs, but then again I'm a true psychonaut. I like to explore and sometimes a bit of a risk is even worth it for me, because someone has to be willing to explore new methods.

Now, I've discussed the combination of many different drugs, potentially mixed with muscimol most of them, but what about combining both "magic mushrooms"; Amanita muscaria and Psilocybe cubensis? Or, even the synthetic versions of both? Yes... Like most good drugs (and bad) there is a synthetic version of psilocybin (the active psychedelic compound in Psilocybe mushrooms, along with psilocin). If I had to guess, both will be increasing in popularity. In 2021, an article was published in the NLM titled; "Homebrewed psilocybin: can new routes for pharmaceutical psilocybin production enable recreational use?".

LSD too, has synthetic alternatives. One that comes to mind for me, is a relatively new drug called 25i-nbome (first synthesized in 2003). Now, I've taken this drug before back when you could order it online legally. It was available on blotter paper, and much cheaper than typical LSD hits at the time. But... to an experienced LSD enthusiast like myself, I could tell the difference immediately. The best way I can describe it, was it felt like more of an artificial chemical-producing high.

Many people say the same thing when comparing either magic mushrooms to LSD, which the user usually describes as more of a natural feeling from mushrooms. So basically that, only amplified greatly. Also, the drug seems to have some pretty serious adverse side effects, and was subsequently made illegal federally. But that's not to say there won't be another synthetic version of LSD, perhaps even in the near future with all of the renewed interest in hallucinogens.

Much like muscimol, an article was published detailing the synthesis of psilocybin (and psilocin). The "Journal of Natural Products" published the article in 2003, titled: "Concise Large-Scale Synthesis of Psilocin and

Psilocybin, Principal Hallucinogenic Constituents of "Magic Mushroom". And if I'm not mistaken, at least some of the trials being done to treat depression or anxiety etc., have been done with synthetic versions (of both muscimol and psilocybin).

Well, now I'm going down a rabbit hole and going off-topic at the same time, kind of, but it will all make sense with time. Keep in mind, I'm trying to explain some very complex things, and tie the information all together in an original and unique way. With that being said, sometimes I have to discuss one topic to be reminded of another, or one topic will lead into another.

However, I am really trying to make all of this information make sense to the reader, and also be easy to go back and find certain sections throughout the book as needed. I'm also extremely excited discussing this topic, admittedly, so I want to make sure I cover it all and don't jump the gun on anything — at least not intentionally.

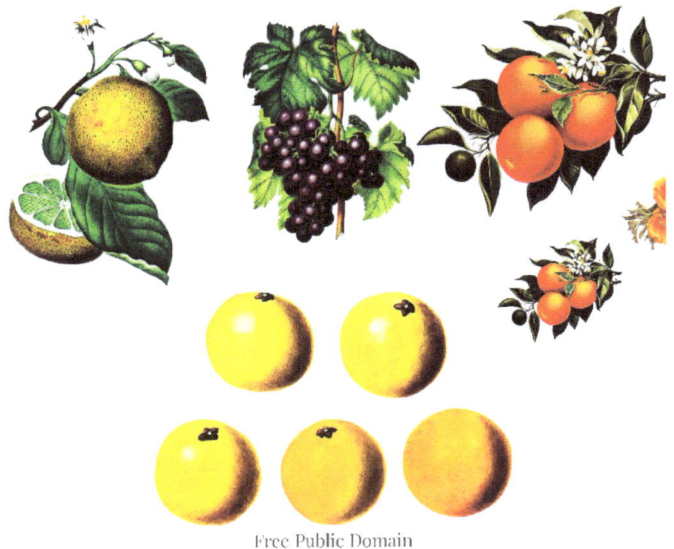

Free Public Domain
Images from Rawpixel
New York Public Library/U.S. Department of
Agriculture Pomological Watercolor Collection

So I'd hate to go back and forth, but I'd like to go back to part of the main topic, which is synergistic interactions (especially relating to drugs). So citrus seems to be another, with citrus likely amplifying many drugs you "take orally", according to the FDA. This is why with some medications you'll be advised to avoid things like grapefruit (and grapefruit juice) and similar products like orange juice (which I mentioned earlier in regards to LSD).

I'm not sure how many of you reading this are fans of Hunter S. Thompson, but surely you've heard of him (hopefully so, one of the greatest writers of all-time) and his book "Fear and Loathing in Las Vegas". Well in that book, and throughout his life as far as I'm aware, he seemed to really enjoy grapefruit. Maybe he knew all along? After all, he did know of what he referred to as "thorazine" when his attorney took too much LSD and he hoped he had some to, what seems like, help him come down from the trip. This would make sense considering there were studies done in the early 1960s about a compound called "Chlorpromazine" and the effects of blocking LSD. "Thorazine" is the brand name of "Chlorpromazine" according to the "Cleveland Clinic".

So, speaking of Las Vegas, let's stay on the desert topic for just a moment. I never hear much about peyote [mescaline] being used synergistically, now that would be interesting. I'd like to imagine the ultimate psychonaut concoction, looking something like; ayahuasca, DMT, marijuana, MDMA, psilocybin, muscimol, mescaline and tobacco all being combined. Could a human handle all of that psychedelic power, all at once? I wouldn't dare recommend it, but no harm in wondering. (I will add: Please don't do that).

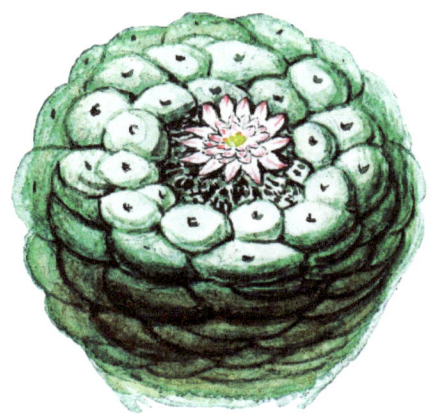

Free Public Domain
Images from Rawpixel
Vintage botanical illustration

So, as I've mentioned previously about
synthetic LSD and muscimol, and yes
mescaline too has a synthetic version. It's part
of the same family as the LSD synthetic, with
the scientific name being NBOMe-mescaline".
If you're a hard-core psychonaut, you may
have heard the slang term "n-bomb" being
used to describe either the synthetic mescaline
or LSD, but more commonly LSD. I've never
taken mescaline (or the synthetic version),
though I would like to experiment a bit with the
drug.

But, I don't want to stray too far off topic (again). So instead, I'll discuss another cannabinoid for now. I think HHC is a good new one to cover. According to "PubMD", HHC [Hexahydrocannabinol] is "chemically like Delta-9 THC, but it's a semisynthetic CBD". Interesting, a "semisynthetic" drug you don't see that term everyday. But the compound's striking similarities to Delta-9, is likely the reason why you also see that in many Amanita muscaria products. Also, I believe HHC is naturally occurring at trace amounts.

Another great cannabinoid which also can only be found naturally in "trace amounts", is THC-A [Tetrahydrocannabiphorol]. According to Wikipedia, THC-A has "reported binding affinity" of "33 times" that of "Delta-9". So, I'm sure you can already assume what that potentially means, and that of course is it may be synergistic with muscimol. And of course the theory is, all of these cannabinoids are in fact synergistic with each other. This would make sense, almost like God intended that by lumping them all together in the marijuana plant.

Where I live [Ohio] marijuana just became legal recreationally. But, now our governor is asking for laws to be made surrounding "Delta-8" and likely similar cannabinoids. This falls in line with West Virginia making (if I read the reports accurately) Delta-8, 9 and 10 illegal. This has already passed the State Senate. Many states have and/or will likely follow suit, which goes against the Farm Bill of 2018 that Donald Trump signed into law. So, once again, government overreach on the local levels and beyond.

If you're a fan of these compounds, then it may be wise to stock up while you can — which is exactly what I plan on doing. For me it's truly a double edged sword, because I've become fascinated with these compounds as of recently, while initially dismissing them entirely thinking it was too good to be true. The stuff was so easily and readily available, that I figured there must've been some sort of catch. I was wrong and can admit it. Okay, moving on now.

So perhaps you're curious to learn more about smoking Amanita muscaria, since there is definitely not a lot of professional research done on that topic. Although there are articles about it dating back to at least 2009, and underground forums etc. So the hard-core crowd has given it a go, but not many people would dare to pack a bowl or roll a joint with crushed mushrooms mixed in. I, however, am a true psychedelic explorer (and I don't say that to sound smug, I remain humble and always a learner). But I've even smoked psilocybin mushrooms, so what the hell. These ones definitely look better, if that makes a difference. I even designed my own cigarette package as a joke.

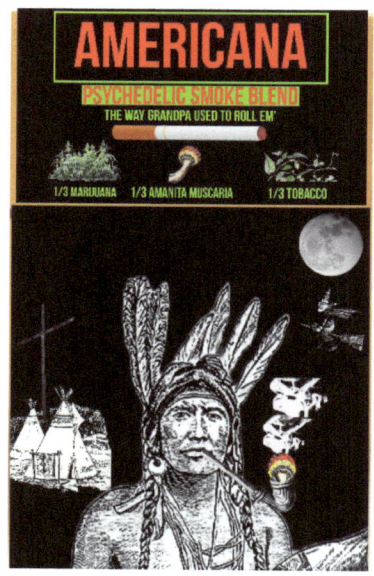

But when I say that I made the package design as a joke, I should say half-jokingly. I 100% stand by that combination as a smoke blend. But of course, my "grandpa" didn't roll them that way, although that is a funny thought, I just thought an old-timey type motto was fitting. But that blend really is a psychedelic smoke mixture, and I usually enjoy that combination by itself, and/or while eating Amanita muscaria + Delta-9 gummies or whatever else I decide to do. I personally thoroughly enjoy the taste, and so do many people I've given it to.

I will say, my preference is actually Amanita pantherina (the brown cap mushrooms) which are significantly more potent and taste more unique. Two hits from a bowl with a dried cap of that mixed, is basically equivalent to maybe six hits of Amanita muscaria (red cap) and of course I'm talking about the combination blend. I rarely eat or smoke the mushrooms individually. Some reports online compare smoking Amanita muscaria to a "weed high", but if they used the combination blend they may just be pleasantly surprised. (If all else fails, eat some grapefruit).

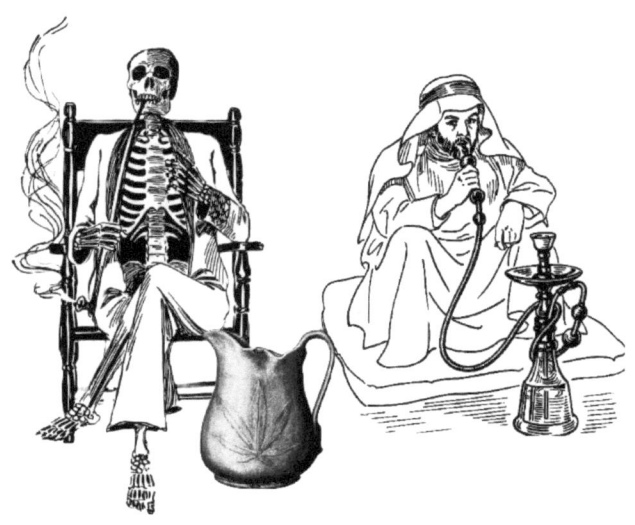

Pitcher (ca. 1938) by Richard Barnett. Original from The National Gallery of Art

Now smoking psilocybin mushrooms on the other hand, at least to me, does give more of a "weed high". While eating marijuana gives more of a "mushroom high" if you will. Now I don't mean exact, just more similar to that of a true psychedelic trip when eating marijuana comaot3d to smoking. Although, marijuana has been (and still is) definitely increasing in potency, regardless of how you consume it. I've had some pretty mild, what I would call trips, from taking too big hits of marijuana. But truly, if I could mix any two drugs, I think I'm going with both types of magic mushrooms. I still have yet to try it.

Really, I have no excuse as to why. I know how to grow psilocybin mushrooms, hell I published a small book in 2020 about it titled "How to Grow Psilocybin Mushrooms: The Complete Beginners Guide to Indoor Cultivation". I also know how to get a hold of Amanita muscaria mushrooms online legally, and/or find them in the wild (at least their varieties in my area). So again I have no excuse, and sooner or later I'll get around to it and report back. But every time I think of the combination of the two, I think of attempting protoplast fusion.

Protoplast fusion is basically creating a hybrid of two different types of plants or mushrooms or whatever you're working with. And if this can be done, then that could be the true key to cultivation. I've floated this idea in a previous book as well. According to a website called "toppr" the process includes "the parent plants are fused together to form a hybrid cell which is cultured on nutrient media". Seems simple enough, yet totally complex at the same time, and that's obviously not the process entirely either. But why not give it a shot, what harm can be done?

In my opinion, the majority of psychedelic research should focus on protoplast fusion with Amanita muscaria and Psilocybe cubensis, and/or another way of cultivation. Whether that be using forest ground cover in a controlled greenhouse-type environment, or special substrate made for mycorrhiza fungi. Or even large-scale controlled outdoor grows, regardless of how long it takes. I thought I found a magical Spruce tree where they would continue to return to me, but I was sadly wrong. But also, the conditions with the mushrooms must be exact.

Magic Mushroom Protoplast Fusion
[Prototype]

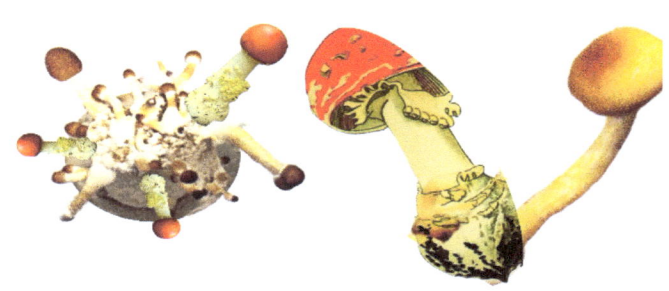

Free Public Domain
Images from Rawpixel
And from Carl F. Miller

But we as humans with so much technology can recreate their growing habitat, can't we? So what's the hold up, has too much time and energy been focused on less important things? One never can be sure, or then again can they? Alright, enough with the rhetorical questions, my apologies. Now, imagine just for a moment (if you will) what a magic mushroom (Amanita muscaria and Psilocybe cubensis) protoplast fusion might look like connected to the roots of a marijuana plant... Personally, I believe where there is a will there's a way.

Another topic in the psychedelic world that always fascinated me was "Psychedelic Telepathy". According to "ResearchGate""40 psychedelics users" participated in a study, in which "16 reported some sort of psychedelic telepathy". As strange as this may sound to some, I've experienced this with LSD. I should also include that I am a twin, and I experienced this phenomenon with my twin brother who was also on it. I could more-or-less read his mind, and vice versa for that matter. It was an extremely memorable and unusual experience for the both of us.

One must also keep in mind, that both Amanita muscaria and (technically Ergotamine, an ingredient in LSD) along with other drugs like black henbane, have a long history with the supernatural, most notably witchcraft.

Examples of this can be found in both; the United States and parts of Europe. So it should come to no surprise that LSD, or "magic mushrooms" are capable of a bit of magic so to speak. If there was no mystery involved, they wouldn't be quite so fascinating to study.

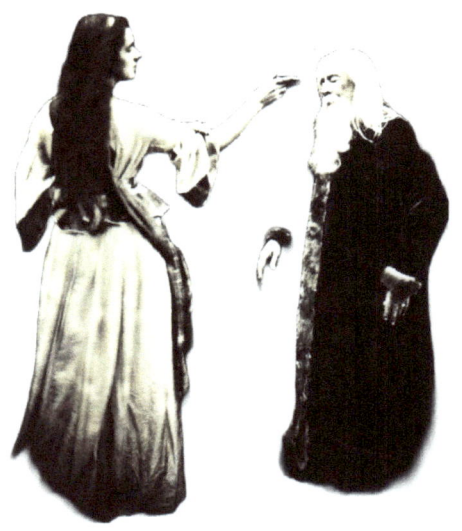

Free Public Domain
Images from Rawpixel
Vivien and Merlin (1874) photography by Julia Margaret Cameron

And just what exactly are you supposed to make of the theory that when you hallucinate on a psychedelic drug, especially something like psilocybin or LSD (or perhaps the muscimol + Delta-9 combination), that all of the geometrical shapes and patterns are what everyone who'd ever taken the drug before you saw collectively? Now that is not a rhetorical question, I'm genuinely curious. I have a feeling that we've yet to hit the tip of the iceberg in terms of psychedelic research.

One guy who stands out today who deserves a ton of credit for his continued psychedelic research, is Hamilton Morris. His YouTube video on Amanita muscaria was the first time I saw someone smoke the mushrooms, and Morris wrote a great article about a drug derived from muscimol; gaboxadol. The article was published in 2013 by Harper Magazine. However promising a muscimol-derivative may sound, I will quickly point out the drug itself was discontinued in 2007 after safety concerns (which I believe Morris highlights in his article).

Morris was ahead of his time covering this drug in 2013, as evident by merely six years later a patent being secured by three inventors for the "Combination of gaboxadol and lithium for the treatment of psychiatric disorders", according to patents.google. There have also been studies about the synergistic effects of the muscimol-derivative. Two of the three inventors secured another patent once again in 2019 as well for the drug. Furthermore, gaboxadol appeared in the news once again in 2023, when "Labiotech" published an article titled; "Drug repurposing emerges as viable option for rare disease treatment", which speaks of the synergistic effects of gaboxadol with another drug [sulindac].

Moving on, I decided to go to "ClinicalTrials" website to see if there were any active trials for muscimol, and to my surprise there was not. Only two trials appeared, one was withdrawn and the other was terminated. Same for Delta-9, no active trials. LSD on the other hand, seems to be in full-swing and multiple trials are actively recruiting, some for healthy individuals also. I should also note that many said trials are being conducted in Switzerland.

Oddly enough, the prodrug to muscimol [ibotenic acid] also has a derivative, a synthetic one, at least according to the NLM in an article published in 1998 titled "Synthesis and pharmacology of N-alkylated derivatives of the excitotoxin ibotenic acid". But I should also note that ibotenic acid is a neurotoxin which most people would generally recommend decarboxylating into muscimol, although perhaps that too would be technically possible (I would assume) with the synthetic derivative.

Muscimol and ibotenic acid both belong to a unique class of compounds called "Isoxazole". According to the NLM, some "marketed drugs", such as "valdecoxib, flucloxacillin, cloxacillin, dicloxacillin, and danazol" also contain these compounds. The NLM also says that "Isoxazole" are the most popular "heterocyclic compounds" for developing "novel drug candidates". In 2021, they also highlighted studies that suggest "These derivatives [isoxazole derivatives] act as an anticancer agent with different mechanisms".

So, once again, Amanita muscaria and all of its compounds (especially muscimol and ibotenic acid) are playing a much larger role than many realize in not only the recreational drug world, but also the medicinal. So to simplify this, without Amanita muscaria (and/or pantherina) there wouldn't be muscimol or ibotenic acid. Without muscimol and/or ibotenic acid, there wouldn't be isoxazoles. Today, the "drugbank" website lists more than 65 rows of drugs containing isoxazoles, now that's pretty incredible.

In all honesty, I don't know who can look at all of this information and numerous studies (with clear proof of their magic), yet still deny that these mushrooms are indeed "magic". And I'm not using the term "magic" loosely. Another possible huge breakthrough in medicine (and more commonly used in addiction therapy) is "hypnosis" which has been gaining popularity in recent years. Now muscimol is truly a hypnotic drug, and in that sense, in some ways similar to "benzodiazepines" aka "benzos". In 1984, the NLM published an article titled "Hypnotic action of benzodiazepines: a possible mechanism".

Benzos and muscimol mainly differ by the areas in which they bind, yet both are sedative/hypnotic drugs. So I just know that 2024 is going to continue to be interesting for muscimol enthusiasts (despite any possible legal status challenges), I've got a great feeling! And although we are nearing the end of this great journey which comes in the format of a book, don't stop reading quite yet. As I still have a conclusion to form.

Conclusion

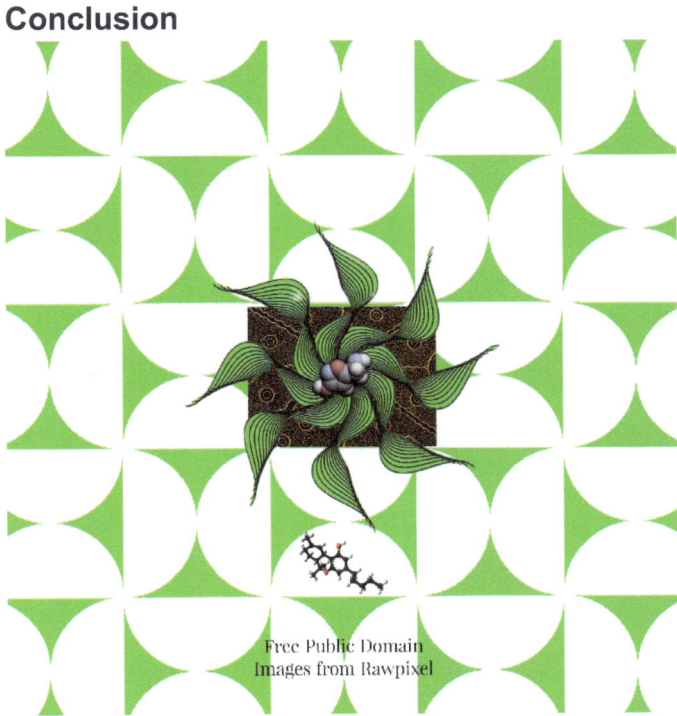

Now, in conclusion I'll touch a bit more on the expected effects, or at least from my standpoint, as well as a few other topics. The combination of muscimol and Delta-9 and/or other cannabinoids, results in intoxicating effects that, to me, resemble psilocybin greatly. And in turn, also resemble the effects of LSD. So I will go on record and say that with the combination involved, that I'd place these mushrooms right up there (in terms of effects) with some of the great, more widely used psychedelics. For me, similar geometrical shapes and patterns were very visible as they were with LSD or psilocybin, with always a shade of either lime or neon green.

Now, I'll always be biased towards psilocybin mushrooms, as in many ways my journey into this incredible world of psychedelics began with them. At least in terms of the first types of hallucinogenic drugs that I've written about in-depth. I began as a small-time psilocybin mushrooms cultivator, then as I learned and improved and tried new techniques, I would document everything in a journal. Then, the journal continued to grow to the point I had enough material for a small book.

I began writing the book [How to Grow Psilocybin Mushrooms: The Complete Beginners Guide to Indoor Cultivation] in 2014 (originally as notes for myself for future grows). I would later publish the book in 2020 for what I deemed a very reasonable price of $6.99 for the paperback. However, psilocybin mushrooms have a lot of people conducting research and documenting findings etc. So I wanted to travel down the road a little less traveled, for lack of a better term.

To highlight what I mean, remember when I mentioned earlier that muscimol only had two trials (both inactive) on the "ClinicalTrials" website that was listed? Well, psilocybin for example, has 161 studies total listed on that same site, with many active. So it's just a completely different amount of research when comparing the two "magic mushrooms". I feel like many people have dismissed Amanita muscaria all together as being "magic", and that is a true shame.

I still see a bright future for Amanita muscaria mushrooms, as last year I described their future as being "almost as bright as their unique colored caps". So this year, which will hopefully be a great 2024, I will modify that quote and say their future will be even brighter than the color of their caps. In the near future, do see these mushrooms being cultivated indoors, as well as a hybrid mushroom being created through protoplast fusion. I also can see clinical trials coming back, and many more studies conducted. But with all of that attention, I also see something coming that I don't like.

What I'm referring to, is the legal status of these mushrooms, and more importantly muscimol. As of this writing, I'm only aware of

Louisiana making Amanita muscaria use illegal (in the U.S). But that can change, and very fast as we are now seeing with the different cannabinoids like Delta-8 and 9. A writer for "leafly" published an article online calling them the "Delta-8 of mushrooms", which may bring more attention right when many states are trying to crack down on Delta-8. But I guess I'm partially guilty too, by further highlighting their psychedelic potential. However, I still feel it's important to document.

In 2023, a website called "LegalScript" published an article titled; "Problematic Products Spotlight: Amanita muscaria". Similarly, a website called "HealthNewsFlorida" also published an article in 2023, which was titled; "Mood-altering mushroom sales bloom despite safety concerns". The "mushrooms" discussed were of course Amanita muscaria. This falls in line with about 90% of articles I read about poisonous mushrooms, which typically have Amanita muscaria as the main image for the article. Stigma like this, will be hard to overcome, regardless of their products popping up in grocery stores.

Another thing I wanted to mention, which in many ways is hard to ignore, is these Amanita muscaria "guru" type people. Now, I know the old saying about minding your own business, and as Hank Williams might say then you "won't have time to be minding mine". But, I just can't stand the idea that you have to go through a specific person for an experience that historically had nothing to do with them. Many of them want to be modern-day shamans, but that is not necessary.

Furthermore, another new cannabinoid that was isolated in 2020, "THC-H". A website called "Delta8us" states that THC-H is "25 times more potent than regular THC", while a separate website [acslab] states that THC-H is "notably stronger than Delta-9". Now that is amazing, but the most potent cannabinoid is supposedly THC-P; which many websites claim the cannabinoid is at least thirty times more potent than Delta-9.

Well, if that isn't good enough news, there is a bit more I will add in closing. There is a website named "analyticalcannabis" that published an article on May 15, 2023 titled; "The New Cannabis? Scientists Find Cannabinoids in South African "Woolly Umbrella" Plant". However this was just one of several new discoveries of cannabinoids in plants other than cannabis plants.

I believe the same can be said for muscimol, because I read an article published by the NLM where they list Tricholoma muscarium as another muscimol-containing species of mushrooms. Amanita gemmata, Amanita regalis and Amanita multisquamosa are all rumored to contain muscimol (and/or the prodrug ibotenic acid). Nevertheless, when it comes to the "Amanita" genus I wouldn't get too experimental, as they also have some of the most deadly mushrooms in the world in that family.

Something else that caught my interest, was I've read two separate people either claim or questioned whether "Panaeolus campanulatus" contain muscimol; one was a user on the website "shroomery", and the other was on a website named "slideplayer". So I'm not sure what they're basing this off of, as I could not find any proof. But if true, this could serve as stepping stones towards protoplast fusion (as more than a dozen species in the "Panaeolus" genus contain psilocybin). Well... I think that's about it. I covered what I've set out to. Thank you very much for reading, I hope you enjoyed it! **The End**

Similar Books From The Author
If you're interested in some of my other books that
relate to this one, then I have several more to
choose from. A few I've mentioned previously, but
I'll go into a bit of detail on each in leaving.

How to Grow Psilocybin Mushrooms: The
Complete Beginners Guide to Indoor Cultivation
is a simple guide to cultivating your very own
magic mushrooms (Psilocybe) indoors, preferably
in a small area like a closet. I give a very deep, yet
simple, breakdown that can turn an amateur grower
into a pro in one read. No images included because
I wanted to keep this book cheap, which I
accomplished with the ebook for $2.99 and the
paperback for only $6.99. Thus, making it one of (if
not the cheapest) books on growing magic
mushrooms.

The Legal Magic Mushrooms of North America:
A Study of the Amanita muscaria Varieties is a
book where I primarily focus on Amanita muscaria
var guessowii mushrooms that grow in the eastern
United States, but also historic use if the
mushrooms in North America and their effects
when compared to classic Amanita muscaria. This
book has some really nice color images so the price
is $10.99 for the paperback, but still $2.99 for the
ebook.

Amanita muscaria: The Ritualistic Magic Mushrooms in this book I highlight dosage expectations, the history of ritualistic use American Indians, new patents, radioactive fungi, different species and plenty of more studies etc. This book is similarly priced (because of a lot of really cool color images, the cost of printing is significantly higher) so again $2.99 for the ebook and $10.99 for the paperback.

The Semi-Legal Mind-Altering Flora and Fauna Handbook: A Guide to Lawful Psychoactive Plants, Fungi, Fish, Amphibians, Reptiles and Insects in this book, I highlight nearly every legal psychedelic drugs and/or loopholes to make them legal in some way or another. Whether this is religious exemptions or participating in clinical trials, or even isolating new compounds from old drugs. This was what I considered my masterpiece in the drug world, yet the book has barely sold any copies (due to me marking the book as adult content during its initial release, not realizing how that would affect sales, do to "adult content" typically being aimed at books containing nudity, which it did not have. Nevertheless, a simple mistake on such a great book). This book is $2.99 for the ebook, $14.99 for the paperback and $21.99 for the hardcover edition.